Ditch The Diet:

Essential Habits To Stay Healthy

By

SHARON BARTON

Table Of Contents

Introduction

Diets, understandably, have taken center stage in our lives in a world obsessed with instant gratification and quick fixes. We are bombarded with commercials for the latest fad diets.

In "Ditch The Diet: Essential Habits To Stay Healthy," you'll discover the stunning truth about the diet industry's web of deception. Prepare for an exciting voyage as you discover the unseen facts that have kept you stuck in a cycle of frustration and disappointment. With a forceful call to action, this book exposes the dishonest side of fad diets and provides you with the skills you need to reclaim control of your health. Break free from the shackles of deprivation, unleash the power of essential habits, and embark on an exciting journey toward long-term wellness. Now is the moment to take action.

GRAB YOUR COPY NOW.

Chapter 1

How To Check Fitness And Health Goals

Goals for fitness and health are crucial in numbers .They urge us to push through momentary suffering to molesting changes, keep us accountable, and broaden our notion of what is possible. But establishing fitness objectives that you'll genuinely want to achieve might be a combination of art and science.

The single objective at a time

Maybe you want to spend at least eight hours at night sleeping, go to the gym every day, and avoid added sugar. That much at once is asking for the family to try to accomplish it. With so many objectives to fulfill, this can result in self-talk that decreases your odds of completing any of the objectives.

Instead, focus all of your energy on attaining one goal—such as mastering the pull-up or running your first 5-K—before moving on to the next.

Recognize the motivation behind your aim.

It's important to address these issues rather than assuming that reaching your goal will make them go away because sometimes fitness goes. Sometimes by underlying fears, insecurities, or body image issues, such as wanting to run a marathon because you were bullied in the middle. After all, enrolling in a CrossFit class because an ex once remarked on your weight.remarked known

Images of the exceptionally fit can make it simple to feel motivated yet envious as you go through social media. However, basing your objectives on what you see others accomplishing is neither useful nor helpful.

Your objective shouldn't be someone else's; it should be something you individually feel enthusiastic about and confidently capable of achieving.

Make it time-bound, precise, and measurable.

A measurable goal enables you to monitor your progress, and the clearer your goal is, the easier it will be to get there.

Prioritize your objectives.

It's crucial to order your objectives according to what matters to you the most. Choose which objectives are urgent and need your immediate attention, and which can wait. Some may be long-term objectives that you may complete gradually. You can more efficiently direct your efforts and energy by prioritizing your goals.

Make a plan of attack.

It's crucial to make a plan for achieving your new goals after you've set them. Your ambitions should be broken down into smaller, more attainable steps or milestones. Make a calendar and plan for your workouts that are in line with your goals, taking into account elements like the type of exercise, frequency, and duration. Create a nutrition plan that supports your objectives as well to make sure you're eating a healthy, balanced diet.

Be adaptable in how you define success.

Though it's crucial to be clear with your goals, you should also allow yourself to change them as you go on your fitness journey. Perhaps a goal that at first appeared to be sufficiently difficult is too difficult to maintain. Moving the goalposts as you get more at ease with your body's capabilities is perfectly acceptable.

Over time, objectives may change and evolve. Keep an open mind when it comes to modifying and adapting your goals as you go along and as things change.

Follow your development

Keeping track of your progress will help you stay inspired and responsible. You can keep track of your workouts, eating habits, and any other important elements using a variety of tools, including a fitness app, a notebook, or a wearable gadget. Regularly evaluate your results and, if necessary, revise your strategy.

Consider a support network.

When considering your objective, you should also consider the people in your life who could inspire you, drive you, and hold you accountable for achieving it. then enlist their assistance anytime you require it. It will significantly impact your life if the individuals you spend the most of your time with support your objectives.

Collaborate with like-minded people, or, if necessary, seek professional advice. Join groups of like-minded people, take exercise classes, or think about hiring a nutritionist or personal trainer who may offer individualized advice and support.

Chapter 2

Power to Lose Weight Frequently

When it comes to reaching weight loss objectives, the importance of habits cannot be understated. You can make long-lasting improvements that support sustained weight loss by adopting healthy behaviors into your everyday routine.

Mindful eating

Practice mindful eating by focusing on your meal, appreciating each bite, and taking your time. This behavior can assist you in identifying fullness, reducing overeating, and encouraging sensible portion sizes.

Take in a lot of water.

Water helps with digestion, keeps you hydrated, and can help you manage your hunger so you can choose healthier foods.

Boost your intake of fruits and vegetables.

Make it a habit to include different fruits and veggies in your meals. They keep you feeling full and satisfied since they are nutrient-dense, low in calories, and high in fiber.

Prepare and plan meals.

Make preparing and arranging meals a regular part of your day. You may make better decisions, prevent emotional eating, and make sure you always have nourishing options available by planning your meals.

Exercise frequently.

Make it a habit to schedule regular exercise throughout your day. Find activities you enjoy doing, like swimming, hiking, or dancing, and set a weekly goal of getting in at least 150 minutes of moderate-intensity activity. The secret to keeping a healthy weight is consistency.

Reduce stress

Utilize stress-reduction strategies, such as deep breathing exercises, meditation, or relaxing activities. Finding good coping mechanisms for stress is crucial because it can lead to emotional eating and impede weight reduction.

High amounts of stress can speed up weight gain or slow down the process of losing weight. Creating healthy coping strategies, such as routine exercise, meditation, deep breathing, or taking up a hobby, can aid with stress management. You can lessen emotional eating and assist your weight reduction objectives by including stress-reducing behaviors in your everyday routine.

Obtain enough rest.

Establishing a nighttime routine and making sure you receive enough sound sleep each night will help you prioritize getting good sleep.

Consistently getting enough sleep can help you lose weight. The regulation of metabolism and the hunger hormones leptin and ghrelin depends critically on getting enough sleep. Lack of sleep can cause these hormones to be out of balance, which can increase hunger, cause cravings, and slow down metabolism. Making a good night's sleep a priority will help you lose weight.

Follow your development

Tracking your food intake, activity, and advancement toward your weight loss objectives should become a habit. To document your adventure, use a smartphone app, journal, or online tool. Reviewing your progress regularly might help you stay regularly for required corrections.

Keep in mind that creating habits requires patience and consistency. Start by making tiny, manageable modifications, then build on them as you go. As you work toward long-term, sustainable weight loss, be sure to acknowledge your accomplishments along the road and practice patience with yourself.

Chapter 3

How To Change Your Mindset for Success

Adopting a positive, growth-oriented mentality that supports your objectives and desires is a necessary step in changing your thinking for success.

Accept that you need to change the way you think.

Everybody has had aspirations and goals that didn't come true the way they were planned or anticipated. When this occurs repeatedly, we begin to question what needs to be altered. But very infrequently we start by changing our thinking from the inside out.

Our culture is skill-driven, emphasizing the development of new skills as well as strengthening our weaker ones. This frequently encourages the idea that we need more education in order tosh our objectives. Some people attend seminars and workshops or study books in search of the magic skill set that will solve all their problems.

Don't get me wrong, I'm not discounting the usefulness of skill sets; rather, I'm saying that more often than not, we need to change the way we think. The good news is that altering your thinking is far cheaper and quicker than learning a new skill.

Recognize your "why"

It takes effort to alter your mentality because established habits are difficult to break. This is particularly true given that many of our most negative routines and mindsets were formed when we were young and have persisted throughout our lives. Understanding your "why" requires a fresh start and the selection of one goal or desire that, when realized, will result in a significant shift in your life. shedding pounds. becoming more content at work. strengthening your bond with your companion. Find anything that might have a big effect on your life.

Adopt a growth mentality.

A growth mindset is a conviction that your skills and intelligence can be improved with commitment and effort. Accept obstacles, view setbacks as teaching moments, and have faith in your capacity to get better and develop through time.

Clear your aims.

Clarify and be explicit when defining your objectives. Put them in writing and divide them into more manageable chunks. This gives you a feeling of direction and keeps you motivated and focused.

Develop self-confidence

Develop self-assurance in your skills and the knowledge that you are capable of achieving your objectives. By concentrating on your strengths and prior accomplishments, you can combat self-doubt and negative self-talk. Do your best to surround yourself with helpful people.

Demonstrate gratitude

You may change your thinking to one's abundance and positivity by practicing appreciation. Consider and express gratitude for your accomplishments, your opportunities, and your supporters on a regular basis, regulates resilience and regularly accepts failure and growth from it.

Instead of viewing failure as a setback, view it as a stepping stone to success. Think about the lessons you've learned and how they can help you go forward rather than obsessing over mistakes or failures. Failures should be viewed as chances for development.

Embrace a proactive mindset and accept accountability for your actions and results. Take the initiative and actively look for answers and possibilities rather than being inactive or reactive. Accept obstacles as opportunities for growth and move decisively toward your objectives.

Surround yourself with uplifting people.

Be in the company of inspiring and motivating people. Find helpful peers, coaches, or mentors who can offer advice and encouragement. Avoid being with toxic people or situations that might impede your success.

Continual education and personal growth

Adopt a lifelong learning philosophy. Look for chances to learn new things, improve your talents, and advance personally.

Keep an open mind and a curious mind, and accept challenges that take you outside of your comfort zone.

Develop your resiliency

Recognize that challenges and failures are a normal part of every endeavor. By overcoming setbacks, adjusting to changes, and being optimistic, one can develop resilience. Consider setbacks as opportunities for development and keep going.

Self-care is important.

Put your well-being and self-care first. Make sure you get adequate sleep, consume a healthy diet, exercise frequently, and schedule downtime for enjoyable activities. A successful attitude is supported by physical and mental health.

Chapter 4

Dietary Supplements

Dietary supplements are an essential component of a healthy lifestyle and can have a significant impact on your overall well-being. Adopting a balanced and satisfying eating plan can benefit your physical health, help you maintain a healthy weight, and lower your risk of chronic diseases.

Take a variety of whole foods.

Take a variety of fruits, vegetables, whole grains, lean proteins, and healthy fats. These foods are high in critical nutrients, fiber, and antioxidants, all of which support excellent health.

Concentrate on portion control.

To avoid overeating, pay attention to portion proportions. Make use of smaller plates and bowls, and pay attention to your hunger and fullness signs. Pay attention to your body's cues and eat until you're satisfied, not full.

Make fruits and vegetables a priority.

Make an effort to fill half of your plate with bright fruits and veggies.

They're loaded with vitamins, minerals, and fiber. To provide a diverse spectrum of nutrients, including a variety of varieties and colors.

Select whole grains.

Choose whole-grain foods like brown rice, quinoa, whole wheat bread, and oats. When opposed to refined grains, whole grains provide more fiber and minerals.

Include lean proteins in your diet.

Incorporate lean protein sources such as poultry, fish, lentils, tofu, and low-fat dairy products. Protein is necessary for tissue development and repair, and it also keeps you feeling fuller for longer.

Reduce your intake of processed meals and added sugars.

Reduce your consumption of processed and packaged foods, which are generally heavy in added sugars, bad fats, and sodium. These foods are high in empty calories and low in nutritional value.

Stay hydrated.

Water is required for a variety of body activities such as digestion, nutrition absorption, and temperature regulation. Limit your intake of sugary drinks and make water your primary beverage.

Limit your intake of saturated and trans fats.

Choose healthy fats such as avocados, nuts, seeds, and olive oil. Reduce your intake of saturated fats, which are found in red meat, full-fat dairy products, and fried foods. Trans fats, which are typically present in processed and fried meals, should be avoided because they can raise the risk of heart disease.

Reduce your salt consumption.

Reduce your intake of high-sodium meals such as processed meats, canned soups, and fast food. To avoid using too much salt, season your dishes using herbs, spices, and other tasty ingredients.

Eat with awareness.

Slow down and relish your meals, focusing on the flavor, texture, and delight of each bite. This allows you to become more in tune with your body's hunger and fullness signals, which helps you avoid overeating.

Because everyone's nutritional needs differ, it's critical to work with a registered dietitian or healthcare expert to create a balanced diet plan that suits particular needs and health goals.

Chapter 5

How an Active Lifestyle and Movement Encourages a Healthy Relationship with Food.

A healthy active lifestyle is a way of living that includes frequent exercise and nutritious eating to improve overall health. It's not about gaining peak performance or elite athlete status.

Nutrition and physical exercise are linked.
Eating healthy foods gives you the energy to live an active lifestyle. Being more physically active can also help to develop knowledge of the body and how food affects health. Physical exercise is defined as any sort of movement that expends energy. Physical activity can help people of all shapes, sizes, and abilities. Some physical exercise is

preferable to none, and the more you do, the more benefits you will reap.

Physical activity and nutritious food supply the body with long-lasting vitality that allows you to meet the demands of daily life. Consistent physical activity increases muscle strength and stamina while also supplying oxygen and nutrients to the organs.

Eating well and staying active have similar benefits on our health, lowering our chance of chronic diseases including diabetes, heart disease, high blood pressure, stroke, and some malignancies, as well as the limitations that come with them.

A healthy connection with food can be promoted by leading an active lifestyle and including regular movement.

Improves general well-being

Physical activity and exercise release endorphins, which increase happiness and decrease stress. We are more likely to make healthy dietary choices that enhance our entire well-being when we are in good mental and physical health.

Improves bodily awareness

Physical activity helps us become more aware of our body's requirements. Regular physical activity can help us grasp hunger and fullness cues better, allowing us to eat intuitively rather than relying on external cues or emotions to influence our eating habits.

Creates a positive self-image

Regular physical activity can boost our body image by demonstrating our bodies' strength, endurance, and flexibility. This positive perspective can diminish the desire to engage in restricted or punitive eating practices while also encouraging self-acceptance.

Increases metabolism

Regular exercise increases metabolic rate, improving the body's ability to use calories from diet efficiently. Knowing that our bodies are well-equipped to handle the energy we consume can help build a balanced approach to eating.

Promotes good digestion

Physical activity improves digestion by encouraging regular bowel movements, minimizing bloating, and overall gut health. A healthy digestive tract allows us to absorb and utilize nutrients from the meals we eat.

Boosts energy levels

Exercise offers us a burst of energy, helping us feel more determined and aware. This enhanced energy can have a favorable impact on our eating choices, prompting us to prefer nutrient-dense foods that provide prolonged energy over quick fixes and processed snacks.

Allows for a healthy emotional outlet

Exercise and movement are wonderful ways to relieve tension, anxiety, and other emotions. Rather than using food as a coping mechanism, being active allows us to channel our emotions into a positive and constructive activity.

Improves overall health

A physically active lifestyle provides various health benefits, including a lower risk of chronic diseases such as heart disease, diabetes, and some malignancies. When we prioritize our health through physical exercise, we are more likely to make eating choices that are beneficial to our overall health.

Enhance with nutrient-dense meals

Eat a range of nutrient-dense foods, such as whole grains, lean protein, fruits and vegetables, and low-fat or fat-free dairy, to provide your body with the resources it requires. Consume fewer foods heavy in saturated fats, added sugars, and sodium (salt).

Reduce your sedentary time.

Reduced inactive time is another essential and simple strategy to enhance health. Sitting during the day, generally in front of screens such as computers or televisions, has significant health consequences that cannot be offset by exercise. Experts recommend breaking up sitting time by standing or walking about for 30 minutes or so every 30 minutes or so.

Create a positive attitude about exercising.

What ultimately helps you sustain an active lifestyle will differ. Recent research suggests that focusing on positive experiences during physical activity, such as enjoyment of movement or perception of energy or strength, rather than outcomes (for example, only focusing on weight loss) can help people maintain a positive relationship with exercise in the long run.

Chapter 6

Understanding the Importance of Sleep

Sleep is vital to every bodily activity, influencing our physical and mental functioning. Our ability to fight sickness, create immunity, as well as our metabolism and risk of chronic disease. Because it affects every element of health, sleep is multidisciplinary.

Sleep is essential for many brain functions, including how nerve cells (neurons) communicate with one another.

Prioritizing good sleep entails developing consistent nighttime habits, creating a sleep-friendly atmosphere, and allocating adequate time for restorative sleep.

Improved memory and performance

Sleep is associated with various brain activities, including:

Memory

Sleep deprivation may have an impact on memory processing and development.

Performance

Sleep deprivation has an impact on people's performance at work, school, and other places. This encompasses concentration, emotional response, decision-making, risk-taking, and judgment.

Cognition

Sleep disturbance may have an impact on cognition by influencing stress hormones.

Reduced chance of weight gain

The relationship between weight growth, obesity, and inadequate sleep is unknown.
Sleep deprivation is linked to increased levels of ghrelin (the hunger hormone), salt retention, and inflammatory markers. It is also emphasized that lack of sleep leads to weariness, which may influence a person's desire or capacity to exercise and live a healthy lifestyle.

Improved athletic performance

Adults require 7 to 9 hours of sleep per night, but recent research suggests that athletes may require more.

Sleep is essential for athletes and those who participate in sports because it allows the body to recuperate. Other advantages include:

improved endurance
more power
improved precision and reaction speed
greater speed
improved mental performance

Reduced risk of heart disease

High blood pressure is one risk factor for heart disease. Getting enough sleep each night assists the body to regulate its blood pressure.

A good night's sleep can also lower the risk of sleep-related diseases like apnea and boost general heart health.

More social and emotional intelligence

Sleep has been linked to emotional and social intelligence. Someone who does not receive enough sleep is more likely to have difficulties identifying the emotions and expressions of others.

Depression prevention

For a long time, researchers have been studying the relationship between sleep and mental health. Insomnia is strongly linked to an increased risk of depression.

Sleep deprivation may cause cognitive changes that increase the risk of depression.

Sleep disruption can also impair emotional regulation and stability, as well as change neurological processes, all of which can lead to depression symptoms.

It improves learning and retention.

Sleep is necessary for memory and learning. Our brains consolidate the information we've learned during the day while we sleep, making it easier for us to recall and retain knowledge. It is especially important for students and others who work on intellectually hard activities.

Improving and maintaining a regular sleep schedule may aid in weight loss and obesity prevention.
Hormone balance and appetite regulation
Sleep controls hormone synthesis, which influences hunger, metabolism, and weight management. Sleep deprivation can upset the balance of

hormones such as ghrelin and leptin, resulting in increased hunger, cravings, and probable weight gain. Getting enough sleep promotes healthy metabolism and can help you maintain a healthy weight.

Reduce inflammation

There is a connection between obtaining enough sleep and lowering inflammation in the body.
Inconsistent sleep, defined as going to bed at different times or waking up at different times each night, might disrupt the body's mechanism of managing inflammation while sleeping.

Improved immune system

Sleep aids the body's ability to repair, renew, and recover. This link extends to the immune system as well. Deep sleep is a reliable source for the body to restore and improve its immune system.

Sleep is an essential, but often overlooked, component of everyone's overall health and well-being. Sleep is essential because it allows the body to rejuvenate and prepare for the next day.
Adequate rest may also aid in the prevention of excess weight gain, heart disease, and sickness duration.

Chapter 7

How to Create a Support System for Your Fitness and Health Objectives

Everyone's support system will be different.

Creating a support network for your fitness and health objectives is essential for long-term success and accountability.

It takes time, work, and nurture to build a support system. Developing relationships with like-minded people who understand your path and provide positive reinforcement will greatly increase your chances of success in reaching your fitness and health goals.

Determine Your Desired "End State" - And Set Achievable Goals

Define your objectives clearly. Having defined objectives, whether it's losing weight, growing muscle, improving cardiovascular endurance, or adopting a healthier lifestyle, can help you convey your demands to your support system.

Look for people who share your values.

Seek out people with similar aspirations and interests. Join local fitness groups, internet networks, or fitness-focused social media platforms. Connect with others who are pursuing similar goals because they will understand your difficulties and provide encouragement.

Involve your family and friends.

Inform your close friends and family about your ambitions and the value of their support. Explain how their encouragement and participation might help your progress. Having family and friends on board can help with inspiration and accountability.

Find a workout partner.

Having a workout buddy can make exercise more fun and accountable. Find someone who shares your fitness goals or is willing to join you on your fitness journey. You can exercise together, share your progress, and provide each other support.

Participate in exercise classes or hire a trainer.

Participating in fitness classes or working with a personal trainer not only gives you expert advice but also exposes you to a supportive community. You can meet people who are passionate about fitness and connect with other participants.

Make use of technology and apps.

Numerous fitness apps and online platforms provide community assistance. Join fitness forums, social media groups, or applications that allow you to interact with others who share your goals and seek advice.

Form accountability alliances.

Create an accountability alliance with someone who has comparable aspirations to you. Check-in on the individual. This accountability method will assist you in staying motivated and on track.

Track and celebrate achievements

Keep track of your development and recognize your accomplishments. Share your accomplishments with your support group, whether it's attaining a weight reduction goal, finishing a difficult workout, or establishing a better habit. Their praise and recognition will boost your efforts.

Communicate your requirements.

Communicate your requirements and expectations to your support system clearly-row they can be you, whether it is with encouragement, healthy food ideas, or joining you for physical activity.

Carry out Violence

You devised a strategy. You have a solid support network. GO HARD NOW, Give it your all, and don't stop till you get there.

Make fitness a top priority in your life. You will most likely have to "cut back" on some of your other activities. There's an old saying that goes, "If everything is a priority, then nothing is a priority." This is especially true in this case; you need to identify everything you're currently committed to daily.